Instructor's Manual for
Epidemiology for Public Health Practice
Second Edition

Robert H. Friis, PhD
    Professor and Chair
    Department of Health Science
    California State University, Long Beach
    Long Beach, California

Thomas A. Sellers, PhD, MPH
    Professor of Epidemiology
    Department of Health Sciences Research
    Mayo Clinic
    Rochester, Minnesota

An Aspen Publication®
Aspen Publishers, Inc.
Gaithersburg, Maryland
1999

Copyright © 1999 by Aspen Publishers, Inc.
A Wolters Kluwer Company
www.aspenpublishers.com
All rights reserved.

Aspen Publishers, Inc., grants permission for photocopying for limited personal or internal use. This consent does not extend to other kinds of copying, such as copying for general distribution, for advertising or promotional purposes, for creating new collective works, or for resale. For information, address Aspen Publishers, Inc., Permissions Department, 200 Orchard Ridge Drive, Suite 200, Gaithersburg, Maryland 20878.

Orders: (800) 638-8437
Customer Service: (800) 234-1600

About Aspen Publishers • For more than 35 years, Aspen has been a leading professional publisher in a variety of disciplines. Aspen's vast information resources are available in both print and electronic formats. We are committed to providing the highest quality information available in the most appropriate format for our customers. Visit Aspen's Internet site for more information resources, directories, articles, and a searchable version of Aspen's full catalog, including the most recent publications: **http://www.aspenpublishers.com**
  Aspen Publishers, Inc. • The hallmark of quality in publishing
Member of the worldwide Wolters Kluwer group.

ISBN: 0-8342-1707-4

Printed in the United States of America

2 3 4 5

*The authors thank Amanda Rust,
graduate student in health science, for her
assistance with the preparation of this manual.*

Table of Contents

Introduction 1

Model Syllabus for Epidemiology Course 2

Chapter 1: The History and Scope of Epidemiology 3

Chapter 2: Practical Applications of Epidemiology 4

Chapter 3: Measures of Morbidity and Mortality Used in Epidemiology 7

Chapter 4: Descriptive Epidemiology: Person, Place, Time 10

Chapter 5: Sources of Data for Use in Epidemiology 13

Chapter 6: Study Designs 15

Chapter 7: Experimental Study Designs 19

Chapter 8: Measures of Effect 21

Chapter 9: Data Interpretation Issues 23

Chapter 10: Screening for Disease in the Community 25

Chapter 11: Epidemiology of Infectious Diseases 28

Chapter 12: Epidemiologic Aspects of Work and the Environment ... 32

Chapter 13: Molecular and Genetic Epidemiology 34

Chapter 14: Psychologic, Behavioral, and Social Epidemiology ... 36

Introduction

This Instructor's Manual provides a model course outline for a semester (15 week) course or a quarter (10 week) course in epidemiology and examples of true-false and multiple choice questions that are keyed to each chapter.

Sample course title:
PRINCIPLES OF EPIDEMIOLOGY

Course description and prerequisites: There is a prerequisite course in introductory biostatistics or statistics. The course covers application of epidemiologic procedures to the understanding of the occurrence and control of infections and chronic diseases, mental illness, community and environmental health hazards, accidents, and geriatric problems.

Expected outcomes: Upon the completion of this course, each student should possess the following types of knowledge:

1. Epidemiology as a tool for assessing potential causal associations, health needs of a population, delivery of services, program planning, and social policy.
2. Assessment of the validity and reliability of such data collection mechanisms as death certificates, patient charts, agency records, and personal surveys.
3. Measurements of mortality and morbidity (rates, ratios, and adjusted rates) and the major sources of error in measurement of disease.
4. Descriptive epidemiology: the amount and distribution of disease within a population by person, place, and time.
5. Research designs such as retrospective (case-control), prospective (cohort), historical prospective, cross-sectional, and experimental (prophylactic and therapeutic trials).
6. Evaluation of screening programs in the detection of disease such as determinants of sensitivity and specificity.
7. Population dynamics and health with respect to the stages in demographic transition and trends in the U.S. population.
8. Epidemiologic aspects of infectious disease (variations in severity of illness, components of the infectious disease process, mechanism of disease transmission, and common source versus propagated).
9. Epidemiologic aspects of chronic disease (multifactorial nature of etiology, long latency period, indefinite onset, and differential effect of factors on incidence and course of disease).

Each student should also develop proficiency in scientific report writing and critique. An example includes the organization of thought and clarity of expression. Other examples are the ability to criticize and assess research published in professional journals, to formulate hypotheses and operationalize concepts, to synthesize research and knowledge, and to set forth a theoretical point of view or conceptual orientation. In addition to the global expected outcomes cited above, specific learning objectives are set forth at the beginning of each chapter.

The instructor may also assign the exercises at the end of each chapter. For example, the "Project: Descriptive Epidemiology of a Selected Health Problem" [p. 153] is a library research term paper project that can be completed during the term. Other exercises provide reinforcement of quantitative skills and specific content areas. They may be completed as written assignments or class discussions.

Model Syllabus for Epidemiology Course

MEETING	TOPICS	OPTIONAL COURSEWORK
1	The History and Scope of Epidemiology	Assignment: Course Overview and Objectives READ: Friis and Sellers, Chapter 1
2	Practical Applications of Epidemiology	Assignment: Study questions in Chapter 2 (homework) Assignment: Media Article Essay (Refer p. 30 #7) READ: Friis and Sellers, Chapter 2
3	Measures of Morbidity and Mortality	READ: Friis and Sellers, Chapter 3
4	Descriptive Epidemiology: Person, Place, Time	Assignment: Exercises in Chapter 4 READ: Friis and Sellers, Chapter 4
5	Sources of Data for Use in Epidemiology	Assignment: Chapter 5 questions READ: Friis and Sellers, Chapter 5
6	Study Designs	Midterm #1 Chapters 1–5 READ: Friis and Sellers, Chapter 6
7	Experimental Study Designs	READ: Friis and Sellers, Chapter 7
8	Measures of Effect	Assignment: Chapter 8 questions (1 and 2, p. 278) READ: Friis and Sellers, Chapter 8
9	Data Interpretation Issues	READ: Friis and Sellers, Chapter 9
10	Screening for Disease in the Community	Midterm #2 (Chapters 6–9) READ: Friis and Sellers, Chapter 10
11	Epidemiology of Infectious Diseases	Assignment: Chapter 11 study questions READ: Friis and Sellers, Chapter 11
12	Psychosocial Aspects of Work and the Environment	READ: Friis and Sellers, Chapter 12
13	Molecular and Genetic Epidemiology	READ: Friis and Sellers, Chapter 13
14	Psychologic, Behavioral, and Social Epidemiology	READ: Friis and Sellers, Chapter 14 Assignment: Class and Chapters Review
15	Course Review	Final Examination (Chapters 10–14)

Chapter 1: The History and Scope of Epidemiology (pp. 1–32)

Note: For all chapters, page numbers in brackets denote textbook location where item is discussed.

True or false questions: Please answer the question true if mainly true, false if mainly false.

T   1. John Graunt is known as the Columbus of biostatistics. [p. 18]

F   2. Socrates popularized the notion that the environment is associated with human disease. [p. 17]

F   3. "Nightmare in Niagara" referred to cancer occurrence among vacationers who traveled to Niagara Falls. [p. 2]

T   4. Molecular epidemiology applies the techniques of molecular biology to epidemiologic studies. [p. 29]

F   5. Most of the time, epidemiologic researchers confront a problem that has a clear etiologic basis. [p. 6]

F   6. The study of brain cancers associated with use of cellular phones would be outside the scope of epidemiology. [p. 25]

T   7. Environmental and occupational health problems are a specialization of epidemiology. [p. 28]

T   8. The Framingham Heart Study, begun in 1949, pioneered research into coronary heart disease risk factors. [p. 25]

T   9. Koch published *Die Aetiologie der Tuberkulose* in 1882, a breakthrough that led to improved classification of disease. [p. 25]

T   10. Neuroepidemiology researches neurological diseases in the population, including multiple sclerosis and Parkinson's disease. [p. 26]

F   11. Short-term cyclic fluctuations in disease rates are less likely to characterize acute infections such as influenza and pneumonia than chronic diseases such as cancer. [p. 14]

Multiple choice questions:

1. The epidemiologic approach is distinguished from the clinical approach by: [p. 8]
   A. Its concern with specific signs and symptoms
   B. Its use of clinical data such as temperature readings
   *C. Its focus on the population
   D. None of the above

2. John Snow, in *Snow on Cholera*: [p. 19]
   A. Was the father of modern biostatistics
   B. Established postulates for transmission of infectious disease
   *C. Was an early epidemiologist who used natural experiments
   D. Argued that the environment was associated with diseases such as malaria

3. Which of the following would represent an epidemiological approach? [p. 7]
   A. Psychiatric case report
   *B. Health survey of a population
   C. Treatment of patient with diagnosed illness
   D. A and C

4. Cyclic variations in the epidemic curve may reflect: [p. 15]
   *A. Seasonal variations in cases of influenza.
   B. That influenza is a disappearing disorder.
   C. Secular variations/trends.
   D. Both A and B

Chapter 2: Practical Applications of Epidemiology (pp. 33–68)

Classroom activity: Most students will have some familiarity with the concept of prevention. Select a topic of public health interest (for example, drinking and driving or teenage pregnancy) and have students propose primary, secondary, and tertiary strategies for prevention.

True or false questions: Please answer the question true if mainly true, false if mainly false.

T 1. Syphilis is an example of a residual disorder—one for which the contributing factors are known but methods of control have not been implemented effectively. [p. 39]

T 2. A dynamic population is one that adds new members through immigration and births and loses members through emigration and deaths. [p. 41]

F 3. According to 1990–1991 data, the firearm death rate is higher in Delaware than it is in Washington, D.C. [p. 44]

T 4. An example of operations research is using epidemiology to plan the placement of health services in the community. [p. 44]

F 5. The National Ambulatory Medical Care Survey is a continuing probability survey of physicians who practice in public settings such as VA centers. [p. 47]

T 6. Five-year relative survival rates for pancreatic cancer by race/ethnic group are below 20% for both non-Hispanic whites and Hispanic whites. [p. 62]

F 7. Health education programs about the hazards of starting smoking are examples of secondary prevention. [p. 63]

T 8. The Henle-Koch postulates were instrumental in efforts to prove the causative involvement of a microorganism in an infectious disease. [p. 50]

F 9. The criterion of plausibility refers to the existence of a dose–response relationship. [p. 56]

F 10. Doll and Peto demonstrated that the mortality ratios for lung cancer were similar for those who smoked 1–14 and 15–24 cigarettes per day. [p. 57]

F 11. A risk factor that is important for the population is always important for the individual. [p. 60]

F 12. John Cassel argued that the agent, host, and environment triad provided an adequate explanation for chronic diseases of non-infectious origin. [p. 52]

T 13. In less developed regions, triangular population distributions are linked to high mortality among younger age groups. [p. 39]

F 14. The existence of a dose-response relationship, that is, an increase in disease risk with an increase in the amount of exposure, does not support a view that an association is a causal one. [p. 56]

Multiple choice questions:

Indicate the level of prevention (A, B, C, or D) that is represented by questions 1 through 5. [pp. 63–64]

    A. Primary Prevention Active
    B. Primary Prevention Passive
    C. Secondary Prevention
    D. Tertiary Prevention

D 1. Half-way houses

A 2. Nutritional counseling for pregnant women

C 3. Screening for breast cancer

B 4. Pasteurization of milk

A 5. Immunization against rubella

6. The uses of epidemiology include: [p. 34]
   A. Search for determinants (causes of disease)
   B. Estimation of individual risks and chances of contracting disease
   C. Evaluation of health services
   *D. All of the above

7. What factors should be considered in measuring true long-term changes in mortality rates due to a specific disease? [p. 36]
   A. Changes in diagnostic criteria
   B. Changes in the age distribution
   C. Changes in the sex distribution
   *D. All of the above

8. According to the natural history of disease model, the time before the precursors of disease and the host interact is called the period of: [p. 63]
   *A. Prepathogenesis
   B. Pathogenesis
   C. Primogenesis
   D. B and C

9. Using epidemiology for operational research involves: [p. 44]
   *A. Study of community health services
   B. Study of risks to the individual
   C. Study of disease syndromes
   D. All of the above

10. The following two population distributions are for: [p. 38]

The Horizontal Axes Refer to the Percent of Population in Each Age Category

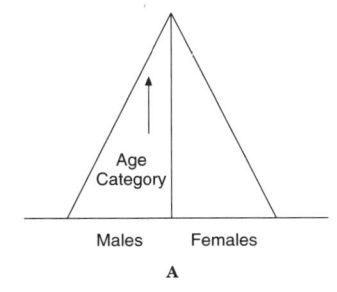

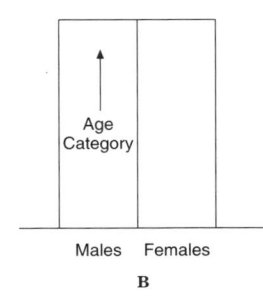

   *A. A = less developed countries, B = more developed countries
   B. A = more developed countries, B = less developed countries
   C. none of the above

11. Which of the forms of prevention takes place after the precursors of disease interact with the host? [p. 63]
    A. Tertiary
    B. Secondary
    C. Primary
    *D. Both A and B

12. Increases in lung cancer mortality, especially among women, illustrate which of the following trends in disease occurrence? [p. 39]
    A. A residual disorder
    *B. A new epidemic disorder
    C. A persistent disorder
    D. A disappearing disorder

13. There has been an increase in the number of epidemiologic studies reported in medical journals because: [p. 35]
    *A. They interest the public and physicians concerned with preventive medicine.
    B. Infectious diseases are predominant in American society.
    C. It is relatively easy to investigate risk factors through experiments.
    D. All of the above

14. The difference between primary and secondary prevention of disease is: [pp. 63–64]
    A. Primary prevention means control of causal factors, while secondary prevention means control of symptoms.
    B. Primary prevention means control of acute disease, while secondary prevention means control of chronic disease.
    *C. Primary prevention means control of causal factors, while secondary prevention means early detection and treatment of disease.
    D. Primary prevention means increasing resistance to disease, while secondary prevention means decreasing exposure to disease.

15. In 1900, the death rate per 100,000 population for influenza and pneumonia was 202.2; it was 21.7 in 1986. How much did the death rate decline due to this condition? [p. 58]
    A. 100%
    B. 1000%
    *C. 90%
    D. 9000%
    E. None of the above

Essay question:
1. You are interested in controlling cigarette smoking among young women, aged 15–24. Describe one primary prevention approach and one secondary prevention approach you would use. Convey your understanding of the difference between primary and secondary approaches in the context of your answer.

Chapter 3: Measures of Morbidity and Mortality Used in Epidemiology (pp. 69–106)

Classroom activity: The concept of rate adjustment is difficult for many beginning students to learn. Illustration of direct and indirect adjustment can be turned into a cooperative group learning exercise. Have the students pair up to work through answers together. Show a sample calculation or two, and then have them break up and work on problem solving in class. Bring the class back together and write the remaining answers down (using an overhead projector) with clarification on concepts and rationale.

True or false questions: Please answer the question true if mainly true, false if mainly false.

Questions 1–4: For disease "X,"

T 1. The **incidence rate** of a disease is defined as the number of new cases of the disease over a time period times a multiplier divided by the size of the population at risk over a time period. [p. 76]

T 2. The **crude death rate** of a disease is defined as the number of deaths due to the disease during the year divided by the size of the population at the mid-point of the year. [p. 73]

T 3. The **point prevalence** of a disease is defined as the number of cases of the disease at a point in time divided by the total number in the group. [p. 74]

T 4. The **proportional mortality ratio** is defined as the mortality due to a specific cause during a time period divided by the mortality due to all causes during the same time period. [p. 93]

T 5. At the initial examination of the Framingham study, coronary heart disease was found in 5 per 1,000 men age 30–44, and in 5 per 1,000 women age 30–44. The inference that in this age group men and women have an equal risk of getting coronary heart disease is incorrect because the data are prevalence data and not incidence data. [p. 83]

T 6. When the incidence of a disease is similar to the prevalence, the duration of the disease is short. [p. 81]

T 7. When the prevalence of a disease is much greater than the incidence, the duration of the disease is long and the case fatality is low. [p. 82]

F 8. Certain diseases, e.g., the common cold, can occur more than once in a stated period of time. Repeated cases of the disease have **no effect** upon incidence rates. [p. 82]

F 9. A prerequisite for using indirect age adjustment is that the number of deaths in the study population must be large. [p. 100]

T 10. A prerequisite for using direct age adjustment is that the age-specific death rates in the study population must be stable. [p. 99]

Multiple choice questions:

1. Rabbit City has a rising population of 500,000 robust, fertile males and 450,000 robust, fertile females. If there were 4,000 live births, 3 fetal deaths, and 40 maternal deaths, what is the birth rate? [p. 84]
   A. 4,000/500,000
   B. 4,000/450,000
   *C. 4,000/950,000
   D. 4,003/950,000
   E. 3,997/950,000

2. The risk of acquiring a given disease during a time period is best determined by: [p. 79]

Instructor's Manual for Epidemiology for Public Health Practice, Second Edition

A. The mortality rate from that disease in the 0–4 age group.
B. A spot map that records all cases of the disease in the last year.
C. The period prevalence for that disease during the last year.
*D. The incidence rate (cumulative incidence) for that disease in a given period of time.

Questions 3–5: An epidemiological survey of roller-skating accidents in Juneau, Alaska, a city with a population of 100,000, produced the following:

Number of skaters in Juneau during any given month	12,000
Roller-skating accidents in Juneau	600
Total residents injured from roller-skating	1,800
Total deaths from roller-skating	90
Total deaths from all causes	900

3. The crude death rate was: [p. 72]
   A. 90/600
   *B. 90/100,000
   C. 90/1,800
   D. 90/900

4. The cause-specific mortality rate from roller-skating was: [p. 92]
   A. 90/600
   *B. 90/100,000
   C. 90/1,800
   D. 90/900

5. The proportionate mortality ratio due to roller-skating was: [p. 93]
   A. 90/600
   B. 90/100,000
   C. 90/1,800
   *D. 90/900

6. Which of the following terms is expressed as a ratio? [p. 71]
   A. $\dfrac{\text{Male Births}}{\text{Male + Female Births}}$
   B. $\dfrac{\text{Female Births}}{\text{Male + Female Births}}$
   *C. $\dfrac{\text{Male Births}}{\text{Female Births}}$
   D. A and B

7. Which of the following terms is expressed as a proportion? [p. 70]
   A. $\dfrac{\text{Male Births}}{\text{Female Births}}$
   *B. $\dfrac{\text{Female Births}}{\text{Male + Female Births}}$
   C. $\dfrac{\text{Female Births}}{\text{Male Births}}$
   D. A and C

Questions 8–12: Incidence and prevalence data have different applications in public health. Below is a list of uses for data. Indicate by choosing the appropriate option whether the use is for incidence or prevalence data.

A. This is a use primarily for incidence data.
B. This is a use primarily for prevalence data.
C. This application could apply equally for both incidence and prevalence data.
D. This is a use neither for incidence nor prevalence data.

B 8. For determining workload and planning the scope of facilities and manpower needs, particularly in chronic disease. [p. 74]

B 9. For estimating the frequency of exposure. [p. 74]

A 10. The fundamental tool for etiologic studies of both acute and chronic diseases. [p. 83]

B 11. To express the burden or extent of some condition or attribute in a population. [p. 74]

A 12. To provide a direct estimate of the risk of developing a disease. [p. 83]

13. Successful **treatment** programs that would shorten the duration of a disease primarily affect: [p. 72]
    *A. The prevalence of the disease.
    B. The incidence of the disease.
    C. Both the incidence and the prevalence of the disease.
    D. None of the above

14. The major **disadvantage** of crude rates is that: [p. 73]
    A. They may not allow for comparison of populations that differ in size.
    *B. They do not permit comparison of populations that vary in composition.
    C. They are difficult to calculate from available data sources.
    D. All of the above

15. Blood pressure measurements on adult males 30–39 years of age were obtained in a survey of a representative sample of Twin Cities households. To compare the frequency of hypertension in the white and non-white population surveyed, the most appropriate measure is the: [p. 95]
    A. Incidence rate
    B. Prevalence rate
    C. Race-specific incidence rate
    *D. Race-specific prevalence rate
    E. Race-specific age-adjusted prevalence rate

16. The incidence of a disease is five times greater in men than in women, but the prevalence shows no sex difference. The most likely explanation is that: [p. 82]
    A. The mortality rate is greater in women.
    B. The case fatality rate is greater in women.
    *C. The duration of the disease is greater in women.
    D. Women receive less adequate medical care for the disease.

Essay questions:

1. Different measures of disease are useful to evaluate and assess public health programs and needs in different situations. For each of the following items, (a) which measure would best support your goal, and (b) explain why you chose that measure.

    Measures of disease:
    I = incidence rate (p. 77)
    P = prevalence (p. 73)
    C = case fatality rate (see p. 349)
    M = mortality rate (crude death rate) (p. 72)
    A = absolute # of cases (counts) (p. 70)

    A. To demonstrate that railroad crossings need to be safer to prevent car-train crashes.
    B. To demonstrate that a primary prevention program is successful.
    C. To demonstrate that a new leukemia treatment is successful.
    D. To estimate the health care facilities needed to support Alzheimer's patients.
    E. To argue that AIDS is a serious public health problem.
    F. To argue that heart disease should get more funding than AIDS.
    G. To demonstrate that a new screening program for breast cancer is effective.

2. Researchers have been trying to gauge the impact of the "Graying of America." They report that currently 5% of the US population is over age 75, and in ten years it is expected that 15% of the US population will be over age 75.
    A. Do you expect that this shift in age composition will result in shifts in mortality rates? Why or why not?
    B. How will you evaluate time trends in mortality rates? Be specific and provide examples.

3. How many people would be needed in order to accumulate 900 person-years of observation in each row? [p. 81]

Number of people	Average time at risk per person
_____	1 year
_____	2 years
_____	3 years
_____	10 years

Chapter 4: Descriptive Epidemiology: Person, Place, Time (pp. 107–154)

Classroom activity: Rather than provide a lecture filled with examples of descriptive epidemiology, here's a technique that will get the class involved and allow them to apply the material in the book. One approach is to have the students pair up and work together to "brainstorm" on responses. Begin by soliciting from the class 2 to 3 topics of public health significance. Then, tell the class to write down 3–5 aspects of PERSON that would characterize this problem. As you get answers from the "groups," summarize by pointing out some are factors easily assessed through questionnaires, others may be available from medical records, and others still may require clinical evaluation or laboratory testing. As descriptors are provided, ask the students what hypotheses they raise about the etiology. Repeat for place and time.

True or false questions: Please answer the question true if mainly true, false if mainly false.

T 1. One of the main purposes of descriptive epidemiology is to aid in the creation of hypotheses. [p. 109]

T 2. The major categories of descriptive epidemiologic variables are person, place, and time. [p. 108]

F 3. Socioeconomic status is an example of a place variable. [p. 126]

T 4. Repeated cross-sectional surveys may underestimate past smoking behavior of older age cohorts. [p. 143]

F 5. The biological clock phenomenon is linked to place variation in diseases. [p. 108]

F 6. Developmental problems such as congenital birth defects occur primarily late in life. [p. 114]

F 7. In the United States, lung cancer is the leading cause of cancer deaths among males, and breast cancer is the leading cause of cancer deaths among females. [pp. 116–117]

T 8. Lung cancer is the leading cause of cancer deaths among both males and females in the United States. [pp. 116–117]

T 9. Marriage is hypothesized to act as either a selective or a protective factor in health. [p. 119]

F 10. Numerous epidemiological studies have indicated that race does not influence the incidence and prevalence of disease. [p. 120]

T 11. The HHANES was a major study of health of Latinos in the United States. [p. 123]

T 12. Nativity refers to place of origin of an individual. [p. 123]

T 13. Religious identification tends to be an aspect of racial or ethnic identification. [p. 119]

F 14. Hollingshead and Redlich found that severe mental illness was more common in the upper than in the lower social classes. [p. 128]

F 15. Infant mortality rates are higher in the upper social classes than in the lower social classes. [p. 129]

F 16. The OECD is a major source of information about international variations in rates of disease. [p. 130]

F 17. Vampire bat rabies increased in the 1980s as a cause of human mortality in the United Kingdom. [p. 131]

T 18. Prevalence of multiple sclerosis varies according to latitude in the United States. [p. 134]

T 19. Temporary stressors may produce cyclic variations in disease rates due to artificial seasons. [p. 139]

Multiple choice questions:

1. **Mortality** rates by sex in the United States generally show the following sex differences: [p. 116]
   - *A. Males greater than females
   - B. Females greater than males
   - C. Males equal to females
   - D. Males equal to females in the first years of life

2. **Morbidity** rates by sex in the United States show the following sex differences: [p. 116]
   - A. Males greater than females
   - *B. Females greater than males
   - C. Males equal to females
   - D. Males equal to females in the first years of life

3. High rates of mortality from hypertension found among African Americans may be due to: [p. 120]
   - A. Dietary factors
   - B. Exposure to stress
   - C. Obesity
   - *D. All of the above

4. Cyclic variations in the epidemic curve for influenza deaths may reflect: [p. 139]
   - *A. Seasonal variations in cases of influenza
   - B. That influenza is a disappearing disorder
   - C. Secular increases in influenza
   - D. None of the above

5. Failing to account for **age** cohort effects in smoking prevalence may: [p.143]
   - A. Obscure the fact that older cohorts had **higher** prevalence of smoking in comparison to younger cohorts
   - *B. Obscure the fact that there had been a shift in the age of onset for lung cancer toward earlier ages
   - C. Obscure the differences in smoking prevalence for males and females, and by level of education
   - D. B and C

6. Descriptive epidemiology characterizes the amount and distribution of disease within a population to enable the health educator to: [p. 108]
   - A. Test hypotheses regarding **causality** of disease
   - B. Generate testable hypotheses regarding etiology
   - C. Evaluate trends in health and disease within a population
   - *D. B and C

7. The descriptive epidemiologic variable, age, is related to: [pp. 112–114]
   - A. The variation in age-specific disease rates
   - B. The occurrence of chronic disease
   - C. Infectious disease incidence in childhood
   - *D. All of the above

8. Reasons for gender differences in mortality may include: [p. 116]
   - A. Greater risk taking by women
   - *B. Greater frequency of smoking among men
   - C. Higher prevalence of coronary-prone behavior among women
   - D. A, B and C

9. Marital status is an important descriptive epidemiologic variable because it: [p. 118]
   - A. Is associated with high suicide rates among married females
   - B. Is theorized to be a selective factor in health
   - C. Is theorized to be a protective factor in health
   - *D. B and C

10. Studies of nativity and migration have reported that: [p. 124]
    - A. Admission rates of foreign-born persons to mental hospitals were lower than for native-born persons.
    - B. Diseases found in less developed regions are no longer a problem in the United States.
    - C. Immunization programs in developing countries have been highly successful.
    - *D. Some migrants have inadequate immunization status with respect to vaccine-preventable diseases.

11. Which of the following statements most accurately expresses the **downward drift** hypothesis for schizophrenia? [p. 128]
    - A. The conditions of life in lower class society favor its development.
    - B. The conditions of life in upper class society favor its development.
    - *C. The illness leads to the clustering of psychosis in the impoverished areas of a city.

D. The illness is associated with increases in creative talents, which contribute to wealth enhancing achievements.

12. Space and time clustering: [p. 146]
    A. Are of indeterminate significance for rare diseases, because the clusters may occur by chance alone
    B. Suggest common exposure of a group of people to an etiologic agent
    C. Have been shown for angiosarcoma and vaginal carcinoma
    *D. All of the above

13. Substantial international variation in rates of disease are **most likely** explained by: [p. 130]
    A. Differences in diagnostic labeling of the condition
    B. Incompleteness of reporting of conditions, especially in developing countries
    C. Variations in classification and reporting of data
    *D. Differences in climate, cultural factors, and national dietary habits

14. Which of the following reasons might account for **place** variation in disease? [p. 138]
    A. Concentration of racial or ethnic groups within an area
    B. Genetic and environment interactions
    C. Influence of climate
    D. Presence of environmental carcinogens
    *E. All of the above

15. A null hypothesis is most similar to which of the following? [p. 110]
    A. Positive declaration
    *B. Negative declaration
    C. Implicit question
    D. None of the above

16. Which of Mill's four canons suggests that there is an association between frequency of disease and the potency of a causative factor? [p. 111]
    A. Difference
    B. Agreement
    *C. Concomitant variation
    D. Residues

17. Which of the following statements most accurately expresses the **breeder** hypothesis for schizophrenia? [p. 128]
    *A. The conditions of life in lower class society favor its development.
    B. The conditions of life in upper class society favor its development.
    C. The illness leads to the clustering of psychosis in the impoverished areas of a city.
    D. The illness is associated with increases in creative talents which contribute to wealth enhancing achievements.

18. Descriptive epidemiology has the following characteristics: (Circle all that apply.) [pp. 108–109]
    *A. Provides the basis for planning and evaluation of health services
    B. Allows causal inference from descriptive data
    *C. Allows comparisons by age, sex, and race
    D. Is the basis of interpretation of experimental trials
    *E. Identifies problems to be studied by analytic methods

19. The incidence of lung cancer among women is increasing. What factor(s) would most likely account for increased cancer rates? [p. 116]
    *A. Younger women are smoking more.
    B. Older women are smoking more.
    C. Women are smoking less.
    D. Both A and B

Essay question:

1. Describe ten characteristics of persons that are used in epidemiologic studies:

    _____   _____
    _____   _____
    _____   _____
    _____   _____
    _____   _____

Chapter 5: Sources of Data for Use in Epidemiology (pp. 155–186)

Classroom activity: Going over long lists of sources of data can be a rather dry lecture. If your classroom is wired to the Internet, bring a computer to the classroom, fit it to an overhead projector, and explore the electronic database resources together.

True or false questions: Please answer the question true if mainly true, false if mainly false.

T 1. Medline, Toxline, and DIALOG are examples of online databases. [p. 158]

T 2. The Freedom of Information Act exempts release of personal medical data. [p. 160]

T 3. A registry is a centralized database for collection of information about a disease. [p. 172]

T 4. The National Health Survey consists of several distinct programs conducted by the National Center for Health Statistics. [p. 174]

F 5. Health insurance statistics provide a generally representative picture of the health status of the United States population. [p. 176]

Multiple choice questions:

1. What would be the best routinely available source of information on cancer incidence? [p. 172]
   *A. Disease registers
   B. Vital statistics
   C. Special survey studies
   D. Hospital clinic statistics

2. What would be the best source of information on adult and infant mortality? [pp. 166–167]
   A. Disease registers
   *B. Vital statistics
   C. Special survey study
   D. Hospital clinic statistics

3. The best routinely available source of data regarding upper respiratory disease incidence is: [p. 181]
   A. Death certificates
   *B. Reports of absenteeism from work and school
   C. Case registers
   D. Hospital records

4. Which of the following is **not** an important criterion of the utility of epidemiologic data? [p. 157]
   A. The nature of the data
   B. The representativeness of the target population
   *C. The reason the data are collected
   D. The availability of the data

5. Why is **thoroughness** of data collection important to epidemiologic inferences? [p. 158]
   *A. The existence of subclinical cases may lead to underestimation of the magnitude of a problem.
   B. Exclusion of segments of society may hinder identification of high risk groups.
   C. The ability to make general statements regarding the health status of a population is determined, in part, by the representativeness of the sample studied.
   D. At least 10,000 people must be studied before coverage can be considered thorough.

6. Which of the following data sources is most likely to be representative of the general health status of a population? [p. 173]
   A. Hospital outpatient statistics
   B. Absenteeism data
   C. Data from public health clinics
   *D. A morbidity survey of the general population

7. Census data are necessary for accurate description of the health status of the population. The concept of a Standard Metropolitan Statistical

Area (SMSA) was introduced in 1949 to create a unit that would: [p. 183]
- A. Standardize urban and rural areas
- B. Delineate census tracts within cities
- *C. Provide a distinction between metropolitan and non-metropolitan cities
- D. Describe political boundaries of major cities
- E. None of the above

8. Cautious use of information from death certificates is warranted because: [p. 166]
   - A. Certificates are not available for everyone.
   - B. Certificates are often erroneous for date of death and sex.
   - *C. Cause of death may not be correct.
   - D. Autopsy results are not included.
   - E. All of the above

9. The cause of death listed on a death certificate may be incorrect because: [pp. 166–167]
   - A. The cause of death is not known.
   - B. Certain diseases carry a stigma.
   - C. Both of the above
   - D. The ICD code may change.
   - *E. All of the above

10. An abrupt drop in mortality due to a specific disease from one year to the next is most likely due to: [p. 167]
    - A. Incorrect listing of cause of death by the physician on the death certificate
    - B. Incorrect coding assignment according to the International Classification of Disease (ICD) system
    - C. Both of the above
    - *D. A change in the International Classification of Disease (ICD) system
    - E. all of the above

11. The Vital Statistics Registration System in the United States collects data on all "vital events" including: [pp. 166–167]
    - A. Births
    - B. Deaths
    - C. Both of the above
    - D. Fetal deaths
    - *E. All of the above

12. The general concept of a metropolitan area defined by the U.S. Bureau of the Census is known as a: [p. 174]
    - A. Census tract
    - B. Regional planning unit (RPU)
    - *C. Metropolitan statistical area (MSA)
    - D. Primary sampling unit

13. Before utilizing data for an epidemiological study, the researcher must first consider: [p. 157]
    - A. The nature of the data
    - B. Availability of the data
    - C. The external validity of the data
    - *D. All of the above

14. Census tracts are: [p. 174]
    - A. Regional planning units (RPU)
    - B. Cities with populations of 50,000 or more
    - C. Urbanized cities
    - *D. Small geographic subdivisions of counties, adjacent areas and cities

Chapter 6:
Study Designs (pp. 187–232)

Classroom activity: One way to help the students appreciate the differences between the types of observational study designs is to work through, in class, what various measures of exposure and disease frequency, and measures of association, can be estimated from each design. A good approach is to create an overhead with a population-based prospective cohort, one with a multi-sample cohort, one with a case-control study, and one with a cross-sectional study. For each of these, make up some numbers (to fill in the 2 x 2 table), and work through (together or after students have had a chance to try to do on their own) each of the measures of frequency and association that have been introduced in the chapter. Students will quickly see that the population-based cohort design allows for estimation of all measures, but others have various limitations.

True or false questions: Please answer the question true if mainly true, false if mainly false.

F   1. A **cross-sectional** study allows the demonstration of a time sequence. [p. 199]

T   2. Controls are needed in a case-control study to evaluate whether the frequency of a factor or past exposure among the cases is different from that among comparable persons who do not have the disease under investigation. [p. 206]

T   3. In cohort studies, information can usually be obtained on the whole spectrum of morbidity and mortality. [p. 218]

T   4. The relative risk is the best epidemiologic measurement of the strength of association between a possible risk factor and a disease. [pp. 223–224]

Multiple choice questions:

Questions 1–4: As an epidemiologist you are going to investigate the effect of a drug suspected of causing malformations in newborn infants when the drug in question is taken by pregnant women during the course of their pregnancy. As your sample you will use the next **200** single births occurring in a given hospital. For each birth a medication history will be taken from the new mother and from her doctor. [N.B.: These mothers are considered to have been followed prospectively during the entire course of their pregnancy, because a complete and accurate record of drug use was maintained during pregnancy.]

The resultant data are:

Forty mothers have taken the suspected drug during their pregnancy. Of these mothers, 35 have delivered malformed infants. In addition, there are 10 other infants born with malfunctions.

1. The relative risk ratio is [p. 223]
   A. 10
   B. 12
   *C. 14
   D. 16
   E. 18

2. What is the exposure status variable in the study? [p. 219]
   *A. Drug usage
   B. Type of hospital
   C. Obstetrical methods
   D. Malformations
   E. None of the above

3. What is the disease status variable in the study? [p. 220]
   A. Drug usage
   B. Type of hospital
   C. Obstetrical methods

Instructor's Manual for
Epidemiology for Public Health Practice, Second Edition

*D. Malformations
    E. None of the above

4. The number of individuals who both did not take the drug and were not malformed was: [p. 219]
    A. 140
   *B. 150
    C. 155
    D. 160
    E. 170

5. A major advantage of cohort studies over case-control studies with respect to the role of a suspected factor in the etiology of a disease is that: [p. 228]
    A. They take less time and are less costly.
    B. They can utilize a more representative population.
    C. It is easier to obtain controls who are not exposed to the suspected factor.
   *D. They permit direct estimation of risk of disease in those exposed to the suspected factor.
    E. They can be done on a "double blind" basis.

6. Case control studies are among the best ways to study diseases of: [p. 217]
    A. High prevalence
    B. High validity
    C. Low case fatality
   *D. Low prevalence

7. Cohort study is to risk ratio as: [p. 214]
    A. Ecological fallacy is to atomistic fallacy
    B. Genetics is to environment
   *C. Case-control study is to odds-ratio
    D. All of the above

8. The following question is based on the information given below:

   Comparison of mortality rates due to cancer of the uterus in users and non-users of supplemental estrogen revealed: [p. 206; also p. 92]

   Mortality rates per 100,000

	Age 45–54	Age 55–70
Users of estrogen	3.0	17.0
Non-users of estrogen	1.0	6.0

   A valid conclusion derived from the above data concerning mortality among estrogen users is:
    A. The mortality rates for cancer of the uterus are lower in estrogen users than non-users in both age groups studied.
    B. A causal relationship is demonstrated between the use of estrogen and incidence of uterine cancer.
   *C. Mortality from cancer of the uterus rises with age regardless of whether or not estrogen is used.
    D. The mortality rate is lower in non-users than users because the symptoms of uterine cancer are detected earlier in the former group of women.

9. Examples of descriptive epidemiologic studies **do not** usually include: [p. 218]
   *A. Cohort studies
    B. Counts
    C. Case series
    D. Cross-sectional studies

Questions 10–19: A large medical center's oncology program reported an increased number of cases of pancreatic cancer during a certain month. The hospital's epidemiologist leaped into action and decided to conduct a research study on the problem. Tumor registry records were searched to identify all cases of pancreatic cancer during a five-year period; cancer patients were matched with patients treated for other diseases during the same five-year period. All subjects in the study were questioned about lifestyle factors including drinking (alcohol) and tea and coffee consumption. The resulting data are as follows:

DATA

LIFESTYLE VARIABLE	Cancer Patients Men	Cancer Patients Women	Other Patients Men	Other Patients Women
Alcohol	185	120	270	260
Tea Drinking	140	110	230	225
Coffee Drinking	190	140	270	240

Note: Total number of male cancer patients = 200.
Total number of female cancer patients = 150.
Total number of male patients (other diseases) = 300.
Total number of female patients (other diseases) = 300.

10. What type of study is this? [See Chapters 6 and 7.]
    A. Experimental
   *B. Case-control
    C. Intervention
    D. Clinical trial
    E. Cohort

11. Does this study have an exposure status variable? [p. 206]
    A. No
    *B. Yes, lifestyle
    C. Yes, disease type
    D. Yes, sex of patient
    E. Insufficient information to answer this question

12. Does this study have a disease status variable? [p. 206]
    A. No
    B. Yes, lifestyle
    *C. Yes, cancer
    D. Yes, sex of patient
    E. Insufficient information to answer the question

Which number best approximates risk associated with: [p. 212]

Alcohol Drinking

13. Men
    A. 2.11
    B. 0.92
    C. 0.71
    D. 0.62
    *E. 1.37

14. Women
    A. 0.21
    B. 1.37
    C. 2.11
    *D. 0.62
    E. 0.92

Tea Drinking

15. Men
    A. 3.50
    B. 1.37
    *C. 0.71
    D. 2.51
    E. 0.92

16. Women
    *A. 0.92
    B. 1.37
    C. 3.50
    D. 0.71
    E. 3.50

Coffee Drinking

17. Men
    A. 0.63
    *B. 2.11
    C. 0.94
    D. 1.02
    E. 3.50

18. Women
    A. 2.11
    B. 0.94
    *C. 3.50
    D. 0.63
    E. 1.02

19. Which factor has the strongest association with cancer for both men and women? [p. 212]
    A. Alcohol consumption
    B. Tea drinking
    *C. Coffee drinking
    D. The factors show no variation in the association.
    E. Not enough information to determine

20. A five-year prospective cohort study has just been completed. The study was designed to assess the association between supplemental vitamin A exposure and mortality and morbidity for measles. The RR for incidence of measles was 0.75 and the RR for measles mortality was 0.5.

    Which statement is correct? [p. 228]
    A. A cohort study is not an appropriate study design in this case because the association between one exposure and two different outcomes is being considered.
    *B. One of the problems that this study may have faced is individuals lost to follow-up during the five-year period.
    C. A cohort study was not a good design to study this association because measles is a very common disease.

    Regarding the RR reported above, which statement is correct? [p. 223]
    *A. Exposure to vitamin A appears to protect against morbidity and mortality for measles.
    B. Exposure to vitamin A appears to be a risk factor for morbidity and mortality for measles.
    C. Exposure to vitamin A is not associated with morbidity and mortality for measles.
    D. Exposure to vitamin A is a risk factor for morbidity and a protective factor for mortality for measles.

21. Which of the following six types of studies most appropriately characterizes the studies de-

scribed below? You may use each study design more than once, but give only one answer per item. [See Chapters 6 and 7.]
A. Cross-sectional study
B. Case-control study
C. Prospective cohort study
D. Retrospective (historical) cohort study
E. Clinical trial
F. Community trial

F To test the efficacy of a health education program in reducing the risk of foodborne and waterborne diseases, two Peruvian villages were given an intensive health education program. At the end of the two years the incidence rates of important waterborne and foodborne diseases in these villages were compared to those in two similar control villages without any education program.

A You would like to assess the effectiveness and efficiency in delivering health services through your clinic. After selecting a 10% sample of all patient visits during the past six months, you are able to characterize the patient population utilizing your clinic in terms of age, race, sex, method of referral, diagnostic category, therapy provided, method of payment, daily patient load, and clinic staff work schedules.

C You are interested in finding out whether middle-aged men who have premature heartbeats are at greater risk of developing a myocardial infarction (heart attack) than men whose heartbeats are regular. Electrocardiogram (ECG) examinations are performed on all male office employees 35 years of age or older who work for oil companies in Houston. The ECG tracings are classified as irregular or regular. Five years later, myocardial infarction rates are compared between those with and those without baseline ECG irregularities.

E To test to efficacy of vitamin C in preventing colds, army recruits are randomly assigned to two groups: one in which 500 mg of vitamin C is administered daily, and one in which 500 mg of placebo is administered daily. Both groups are followed to determine the number and severity of subsequent colds.

D The physical examination records of the incoming freshmen class of 1935 at the University of Minnesota are examined in 1980 to see if their recorded height and weight at the time of admission to the university are related to their chance of developing coronary heart disease by 1981.

C The entire population of a given community is examined and all who are judged to be free of bowel cancer are questioned extensively about their diets. These people are then followed for several years to see whether or not their eating habits will predict their risk of developing bowel cancer.

22. In case-control studies, the odds ratio is used as an estimate of the relative risk. In order for this approximation to be reasonable, some conditions must be met. Which of the following conditions is **not** necessary in order to use the odds ratio to estimate the relative risk? [pp. 213–215]
A. Controls are representative, with respect to exposure, of the population to which you want to generalize your results.
B. The event (disease) under study is rare in the population.
*C. The exposure in question is rare in the population.
D. Cases are representative of all cases.

Essay questions:
1. Five cases of big toe cancer have been found in the Yukon Territory. Because there are only a few cases, you decide to do a matched case-control study to determine if shoe size larger than 9 is a risk factor for big toe cancer. Cases were individually matched to one control for daily activity, history of athlete's foot, and history of ingrown toenails. The following data were gathered: [p. 214]

Pair	Shoe size > 9 Case	Control
1	Yes	No
2	No	No
3	No	Yes
4	Yes	Yes
5	No	Yes

Compute the proper measure of association. Interpret your results.

Chapter 7: Experimental Study Designs (pp. 233–261)

True or false questions: Please answer the question true if mainly true, false if mainly false.

T   1. A clinical trial entails comparing a group of patients treated with a test treatment to a comparable group of patients receiving a control treatment. [p. 241]

F   2. Intervention studies involve only controlled clinical trials. [p.236]

T   3. Randomized controlled community trials may be used in special situations such as simple intervention studies. [p. 244]

F   4. External validity is not connected with the selection of sample subjects. [p. 257]

T   5. In community intervention studies, it is important for the investigator to quantify and evaluate whether a program has achieved its intended results before assuming the benefits of the intervention. [p. 254]

T   6. A treatment crossover refers to any change of treatment for a patient in a clinical trial that involves switch of study treatments. [p. 246]

Multiple choice questions:

1. Controlled clinical trials enable researchers to: [p. 234]
   A. Derive knowledge about the origins of a disease
   B. Control the level of exposure to a treatment
   C. More accurately identify cause and effect
   *D. All of the above

2. Intervention designs are utilized to explore: [p. 236]
   A. The etiology and natural history of disease
   B. The differences in exposure frequency that may be associated with one group having the disease of interest
   C. The efficiency of prevention measures
   *D. All of the above

3. To assess clinical end points, investigators: [p. 239]
   A. Compare rates of disease
   B. Compare rates of death
   C. Compare rates of recovery
   *D. All of the above

4. The Stanford Five-City Project, a major community trial designed to lower the risk of cardiovascular diseases, used two types of surveys to measure treatment-control differences across risk factors. What were they? [p. 250]
   *A. Cohort and cross-sectional surveys
   B. Community and cross-sectional surveys
   C. Clinical end-point and outcomes surveys
   D. Case-control and cohort surveys

5. A prophylactic trial is designed to: [p. 239]
   A. Compare rates of disease, death, and recovery in a population
   B. Measure how well drugs produce improvement in the patient's illness
   *C. Evaluate the effectiveness of a substance used to prevent disease
   D. Estimate the impact of exposure on the incidence of disease

6. Surrogate end points in clinical trials may include: [p. 240]
   A. Subclinical disease
   B. Physical measures such as the reduction in blood pressure
   C. Reduction is symptoms associated with disease
   *D. All of the above

Instructor's Manual for Epidemiology for Public Health Practice, Second Edition

7. The purpose of double blinding in clinical trials is to: [p. 242]
   A. Reduce error that results from how the outcome is assessed
   B. Reduce error that results from subjects' participation in the trial
   C. Reduce error that results from assignment to study conditions
   *D. A and C only
   E. All of the above

8. Phase III clinical trials for a cancer drug involve: [p. 245]
   A. Initial testing in humans
   B. Testing with different tumor types
   *C. Comparing survival rates among the drug and extant therapies
   D. None of the above

9. The purpose of randomization is to: [p. 245]
   A. Reduce error that results from how the outcome is assessed
   B. Reduce error that results from subjects' participation in the trial
   *C. Reduce error that results from assignment to study conditions
   D. A and C only
   E. All of the above

10. A major advantage of community trials is that they are: [p. 245]
    A. Able to control delivery of the intervention to different study units
    *B. Able to estimate directly the realistic impact of behavior change
    C. Able to randomize subjects precisely to the study conditions
    D. All of the above

11. Which type of evaluation requires the collection of baseline information before the program starts? [p. 253]
    A. Process evaluation
    *B. Impact evaluation
    C. Outcome evaluation
    D. None of the above

12. Which types of health issues are likely to be addressed in community trials? [p. 253]
    A. Smoking cessation.
    B. HIV/AIDS
    C. Healthy eating
    *D. All of the above topics

Chapter 8:
Measures of Effect (pp. 262–280)

True or false question: Please answer the question true if mainly true, false if mainly false.

F   1. The attributable risk is defined as the ratio of the incidence of the disease among exposed individuals to the incidence among non-exposed individuals. [p. 263]

Multiple choice questions:

1. The population etiologic fraction is a measure of the proportion of the disease rate in a population attributable to the exposure of interest. This measure of effect is influenced by: [p. 270, formula 4]
   A. The relative risk of the disease in exposed individuals versus unexposed individuals
   B. The prevalence of the disease in the population
   C. The prevalence of the exposure in the population
   D. A and B
   *E. A and C

2. The population etiologic fraction for a particular disease from Factor X alone is five times greater than that from Factor Y alone. If the relative risk associated with Factor X is 2, and with Factor Y is 20, which of the following statements is true? [p. 270]
   A. The risk of developing the disease is greater in those exposed to Factor X only, than in those exposed to Factor Y only.
   *B. Fewer persons are exposed to Factor Y than to Factor X.
   C. The proportion of the disease in the population attributable to Factor Y is greater than that attributable to Factor X.
   D. More persons are exposed to Factor Y than to Factor X.
   E. The risk of developing the disease for persons exposed to Factor Y is five times greater than for persons exposed to Factor X.

The next four questions are based on the following information:

The death rate per 100,000 for lung cancer is seven among non-smokers and 71 among smokers. The death rate per 100,000 for coronary thrombosis is 422 among non-smokers and 599 among smokers. The prevalence of smoking in the population is 55%.

3. The relative risk of dying for a smoker compared to a non-smoker is: [p. 265]
   A. 9.1 for lung cancer and 0.30 for coronary thrombosis
   B. 9.1 for lung cancer and 1.4 for coronary thrombosis
   C. 10.1 for lung cancer and 8.4 for coronary thrombosis
   *D. 10.1 for lung cancer and 1.4 for coronary thrombosis
   E. 12.4 for lung cancer and 1.7 for coronary thrombosis

4. Among smokers, the etiologic fraction of disease due to smoking is: [p. 268, formula 2]
   A. 0.90 for lung cancer and 0.88 for coronary thrombosis
   *B. 0.90 for lung cancer and 0.29 for coronary thrombosis
   C. 0.89 for lung cancer and 0.88 for coronary thrombosis
   D. 0.89 for lung cancer and 0.29 for coronary thrombosis
   E. Cannot be determined from the information provided

5. The population etiologic fraction of disease due to smoking is: [p. 270, formula 4]
   A. 0.80 for lung cancer and 0.28 for coronary thrombosis

Instructor's Manual for
Epidemiology for Public Health Practice, Second Edition

B. 0.80 for lung cancer and 0.18 for coronary thrombosis
C. 0.83 for lung cancer and 0.28 for coronary thrombosis
*D. 0.83 for lung cancer and 0.18 for coronary thrombosis
E. Cannot be determined from the information provided

6. On the basis of the relative risk and etiologic fractions associated with smoking for lung cancer and coronary thrombosis, which of the following statements is most likely to be correct? [pp. 264–271]
   A. Smoking seems much more likely to be causally related to coronary thrombosis than to lung cancer.
   *B. Smoking seems much more likely to be causally related to lung cancer than to coronary thrombosis.
   C. Smoking seems to be equally causally related to both lung cancer and coronary thrombosis.
   D. Smoking does not seem to be causally related to either lung cancer or coronary thrombosis.
   E. No comparative statement is possible between smoking and lung cancer or coronary thrombosis.

7. If it is accepted that an observed association is a causal one, an estimate of the impact that a successful preventive program might have can be derived from: [p. 263]
   A. Relative risk
   B. Higher life expectancy
   *C. Attributable risk
   D. Prevalence rates
   E. All of the above

SAMPLE 2 x 2 TABLE

	Outcome +	Outcome −	Total
Factor			
+	A	B	A + B
−	C	D	C + D
Total	A + C	B + D	A + B + C + D

Please answer question #8 by referring to the 2 x 2 table above.

8. Assuming that the sample table is for a cohort study, define the risk difference or attributable risk: [p. 263]
   A. (A/A+C) / (B/B+D)
   B. (A/A+B) / (C/C+D)
   C. (A/A+C) − (B/B+D)
   *D. (A/A+B) − (C/C+D)
   E. None of the above

9. When assessing a positive relationship between alcohol consumption and oral cancer using a case-control study, increasing the sample size of the study will result in which of the following: [p. 273]
   A. A lower p value
   B. A greater odds ratio
   C. A smaller 95% confidence interval
   D. A higher disease prevalence

   Circle the best response.
   *1. A and C only
   2. B and D only
   3. A, B, and C only
   4. All of the above
   5. None of the above

Essay question:

1. In a population-based cohort study, an entire community was interviewed regarding smoking habits and then followed for one year. All lung cancer deaths were ascertained and the following data were available:

	Number of individuals	Lung cancer deaths
Smokers	24,500	15
Non-smokers	10,500	2

   A. Calculate the proper measure of association of smoking and lung cancer death. Interpret your results. [Relative risk (RR) = 3.2] [p. 266]
   B. Calculate the population risk difference. Interpret your results. [I_P = 48.6; I_{ne} = 19.1; I_P − I_{ne} = 48.6 − 19.1 = 29.5/100,000 per year] [p. 266]
   C. Calculate the population attributable risk for smoking and lung cancer based on these data. Interpret your results. [29.5/48.6 x 100 = 60.7%] [p. 269, equation 3]

Chapter 9: Data Interpretation Issues (pp. 281–304)

True or false question: Please answer the question true if mainly true, false if mainly false.

T   1. The purpose of matching in a case-control study is to select the controls in such a way that the control group has the same distribution as the cases with respect to certain confounding variables. [p. 295]

Multiple choice questions:

1. In a study to determine the incidence of a chronic disease, 150 people were examined at the end of a three-year period. Twelve cases were found, giving a cumulative risk of 8%. Fifty other members of the initial cohort could not be examined; 20 of these 50 could not be examined because they died. Which source of bias may have affected the study? [p. 289; p. 293, Figure 9–2]
   A. Non-response bias
   B. Hawthorne effect
   *C. Survival bias
   D. Detection bias

2. You are investigating the role of physical activity in heart disease and you suggest that physical activity protects against having a heart attack. While presenting this data to your colleagues, someone asks if you have thought about confounders such as factor X. This factor X could have confounded your interpretation of the data if it: [p. 290]
   A. Is a factor for some other disease, but not heart disease
   *B. Is a factor associated with physical activity and heart disease
   C. Is a part of the pathway by which physical activity affects heart disease
   D. Has caused a lack of follow-up of test subjects

3. The strategy that is not aimed at reducing selection bias is: [p. 292]
   A. Development of an explicit case definition
   B. Encouragement of high participation rates
   *C. Standardized protocol for structured interviews
   D. Enrollment of all cases in a defined time and region

4. Which of the following is not a method for controlling the effects of confounding in epidemiologic studies? [p. 295]
   A. Randomization
   B. Stratification
   C. Matching
   *D. Blinding
   E. None of the above

5. The purpose of a "double blind" study is to: [p. 294]
   A. Achieve comparability of cases and controls
   B. Reduce the effects of sampling variation
   *C. Avoid observer and interviewee bias
   D. Avoid observer bias and sampling variation
   E. Avoid interviewee bias and sampling variation

6. In a survey that uses lay interviewers to interview one person about his health and that of members of his household, the sources of error include: [pp. 292–295]
   A. The person with disease has had no symptoms and is not aware of the disease.
   B. The respondent provides the information but the interviewer doesn't record it or records it incorrectly.
   C. The interviewer doesn't ask the questions which he is instructed to ask, or asks them incorrectly.

    D. The person has had symptoms but has had medical attention and does not know the name of the disease.
  *E. All of the above

7. An epidemiologic experiment is performed in which one group is exposed to the suspected factor and the other is not. All individuals with an odd hospital admission number are assigned to the second group. The main purpose of this procedure is to: [p. 295]
    A. Ensure a "double blind" study
    B. Prevent observer bias with respect to the factor
    C. Prevent observer bias with respect to the outcome
  *D. Improve the likelihood that the two groups will be comparable with regard to other relevant factors
    E. Guarantee comparability of the two groups with regard to other relevant factors

8. A "double blind" study of a vaccine is one in which: [p. 294]
    A. The study group receives the vaccine and the control group receives a placebo.
    B. Neither observers nor subjects know the nature of the placebo.
  *C. Neither observers nor subjects know which subject receives the vaccine and which receives a placebo.
    D. Neither the study group nor the control group knows the identity of the observers.
    E. The control group does not know the identity of the study group.

9. Surgeons at Hospital A report that the mortality rate at the end of a one-year follow-up after a new coronary bypass procedure is 15%. At Hospital B, the surgeons report a one-year mortality rate of 8% for the same procedure. Before concluding that the surgeons at Hospital B have vastly superior skill, which of the following possible confounders would you examine? [entire chapter, pp. 281–304]
    A. The severity (stage) of disease of the patients at the two hospitals at baseline
    B. The start of the one-year follow-up at both hospitals (after operation versus after discharge)
    C. Difference in the post-operative care at the two hospitals
    D. Equally thorough follow-up for mortality
  *E. All of the above

Chapter 10: Screening for Disease in the Community (pp. 305–332)

True or false questions: Please answer the question true if mainly true, false if mainly false.

T 1. **Sensitivity** refers to the ability of a screening test to identify correctly all screened individuals who have a disease. [p. 318]

T 2. **Specificity** refers to the ability of a screening test to identify only nondiseased individuals who actually do not have the disease. [p. 318]

T 3. **Reliability** relates to the ability of a measure to be consistently reproducible, regardless of its accuracy. [p. 314]

Multiple choice questions:

1. Sensitivity and specificity of a screening test refer to its: [p. 318]
   A. Reliability
   *B. Validity
   C. Yield
   D. Repeatability
   E. None of the above

The figure on page 317 represents different combinations and qualities of validity and reliability (high vs. low).

2. Which set of symbols represents high validity? [p. 317]
   A. A
   B. B
   *C. C
   D. Both A and C
   E. None of the above

3. Which set of symbols represents high reliability? [p. 317]
   A. A
   B. B
   C. C
   *D. Both A and C
   E. None of the above

4. Which set of symbols represents low reliability? [p. 317]
   A. A
   *B. B
   C. C
   D. Both A and C
   E. None of the above

5. Which set of symbols represents high validity but low reliability? [p. 317]
   A. A
   B. B
   C. C
   D. Both A and C
   *E. None of the above

6. A set of questions that really measures type A behavior when the theoretical concept desired is life stress has: (Choose the best answer.) [p. 315]
   A. Low predictive validity
   B. Low concurrent validity
   *C. Low construct validity
   D. None of the above

7. The degree of agreement between several trained experts refers to: [p. 314]
   A. Internal consistency
   B. Repeated measures
   C. Concurrent validity
   *D. Interjudge reliability
   E. Both A and C

8. A test that determines whether disease is present is a: [p. 308]
   A. Screening test
   *B. Diagnostic test
   C. Reliability test
   D. None of the above

9. Drs. Poke and Jab (1993) conducted research at all shopping malls in California to detect high blood pressure and to warn people of the potential for hypertension. Their subjects were chosen from those passing by the mall. Which type of program is this? [p. 306]
   A. Selective screening
   B. Mass screening
   *C. Ad hoc screening
   D. Multiphasic screening

Questions 10 and 11: A screening examination was performed on 250 persons for factor X which is found in disease Y. A definitive diagnosis for disease Y among the 250 persons had been obtained previously. The results are charted below:

RESULTS OF DIAGNOSIS

TEST RESULTS	Disease Present	Disease Absent
Positive for Factor X	40	60
Negative for Factor X	10	140

10. The sensitivity of this test is expressed as: [p. 318]
    A. 30%
    B. 70%
    C. 56%
    D. 7%
    *E. 80%

11. The specificity of this test is expressed as: [p. 318]
    A. 30%
    *B. 70%
    C. 56%
    D. 7%
    E. 80%

12. Lead time bias is best described as: [p. 325]
    A. An apparent lower survival among persons screened compared to an unscreened group
    B. An actual longer survival time for persons identified during a screening program because they were given an effective treatment
    C. A similar survival time for persons identified during a screening program relative to persons who are diagnosed by clinical symptoms
    *D. An apparent longer survival among persons identified during a screening program because they were identified at an earlier stage of their disease

13. A new antibody test detects serum antibodies against virus X (sensitivity 99%, specificity 90%). When applied in a group of hospitalized patients diagnosed as having virus X infections, the test is found to have a positive predictive value of 85%. When used to screen a group of "healthy" blood donors for virus X infections, the test is found to have a positive predictive value of 30%. Which of the following best explains this difference between the positive predictive values? [p. 320]
    A. Measurement error
    *B. The prevalence of virus X infection is higher among the hospital patients than among blood donors.
    C. Cases of virus X infection are more severe in the hospital.
    D. Lead time bias occurs among the blood donors.

14. A new blood test has been developed to screen for disease Z. Researchers establish 50 units as a cut point above which a test is considered positive and thereby indicative of disease. The test's manufacturers determine that the test's sensitivity is unacceptably low. However, the manufacturers are not concerned with the specificity and do not want the cost of the test to rise. How can they improve the sensitivity of the test? [pp. 323–324]
    A. Test each person's blood twice
    *B. Lower the cut point below 50 units
    C. Raise the cut point above 50 units
    D. They cannot improve this test and should begin work developing a new test.

15. The adverse consequences of using a screening test that has a low specificity include: [entire chapter, pp. 305–332]
    1. Unnecessarily subjecting people to a potential risk associated with diagnostic procedures
    2. Possible psychological trauma that accompanies suspicion of a disease
    3. Increased burden on further diagnostic services
    4. Increased costs of the screening test

Which of the above statements are correct?

   A. 1, 2 and 3 only
   B. 1 and 3 only
   C. 2 and 4 only

D. 4 only
*E. 1, 2, 3 and 4

16. The conditions favorable to population screening for pre-symptomatic diagnosis of a given disease include: [entire chapter, pp. 305–332]
    1. A relatively high prevalence of the disease
    2. Availability of effective treatment
    3. A screening test with a high degree of sensitivity
    4. Availability of physicians to perform the screening test procedure

Which of the above statements are correct?

*A. 1, 2 and 3 only
B. 1 and 3 only
C. 2 and 4 only
D. 4 only
E. 1, 2, 3 and 4

Questions 17–18: A new screening test for Lyme disease is developed for use in the general population. The sensitivity and specificity of the new test are 60% and 70%, respectively. Three hundred people are screened at a clinic during the first year the new test is implemented. (Assume that the true prevalence of Lyme disease among clinic attenders is 10%.)

Calculate the following values:

17. The predictive value of a positive test is: [p. 320]
    A. 33.0%
    *B. 18.2%
    C. 94.0%
    D. 22.2%
    E. 6.0%

18. The number of false positives is: [p. 320]
    A. 99
    B. 9
    C. 12
    D. 2162
    *E. 81

Essay question: [p. 314]

1. Cataracts of the eye may be difficult to diagnose, especially in the early stages. In a study of the reliability of their diagnoses, two physicians each examined the same 1,000 eyes, without knowing the other's diagnoses. Each physician found 100 eyes with cataracts. Does this mean that the diagnoses are reliable? Please provide a short answer explaining your position.

Chapter 11: Epidemiology of Infectious Diseases (pp. 333–376)

True or false questions: Please answer the question true if mainly true, false if mainly false.

F   1. Colonization refers to the spread of plague to the Americas by settlers from Europe. [p. 344]

T   2. A secondary attack rate is used to show the spread of infectious diseases in a household. [p. 347]

T   3. Aseptic meningitis, viral hepatitis, and tuberculosis are examples of diseases transmitted directly (person-to-person). [p. 341]

F   4. When an individual comes into contact with a piece of clothing that subsequently infects him/her, that piece of clothing is a fomite and the infection is direct. [p. 345]

F   5. Diseases that have only human reservoirs and are transmitted from person to person are the zoonoses. [p. 341]

F   6. Eradication of smallpox was successful because of a program to immunize its primary reservoir, the green monkey in central Africa. [p. 341]

T   7. The term **generation time** relates to the time interval between lodgment of an infectious agent in a host and the maximal infectivity of the host. [p. 343]

T   8. **Herd immunity** refers to protection of a population against an infectious disease when a large proportion of individuals are immune through either vaccinations or past infections. [p. 343]

F   9. The **case fatality rate** is the same thing as the mortality rate for a disease. [p. 349]

T 10. The reservoir for Q fever is infected livestock, e.g., cattle, sheep, or goats. [p. 363]

F 11. Home canned foods would be a likely source for an outbreak of salmonellosis. [p. 352]

T 12. **Vaccine preventable diseases** include *Hoemophilus influenzae* type b (Hib). [p. 360]

T 13. After the introduction of measles vaccine in the early 1960s, the reported numbers of measles cases dropped dramatically. [p. 361]

T 14. Reasons for the resurgence of tuberculosis include the increasing prevalence of HIV infection. [p. 358]

T 15. The largest increase in the number of tuberculosis cases in recent years has been in the 25–44 year age group. [p. 361]

T 16. An **enzootic** disease among animals is similar to an endemic disease among humans. [p. 361]

T 17. Lyme disease is an example of a disease transmitted by arthropod vectors. [p. 366]

T 18. Administration of immune globulin confers passive immunity. [p. 340]

F 19. Physical environmental factors in the natural history of disease include weather, temperature, and biologic components. [p. 341]

T 20. The social environment refers to the totality of behavioral, personality, and cultural characteristics of a group of people. [p. 341]

F 21. Pathogenicity of an infectious agent is measured by the case fatality rate. [p. 337]

T 22. Vectors can be considered as one way in which infectious diseases can be transmitted. [p. 345]

F 23. Incubation period refers to the time between the start of the infection and the beginning of the period of communicability. [p. 343]

F 24. Outbreaks in infectious disease can occur only when there are changes in the host **and** the environment. [p. 338]

T 25. If a disease is fatal, virulence can be measured by the case fatality rate. [p. 338]

T 26. The **case fatality rate** of a disease is defined as the number of deaths due to the disease divided by the number of cases of the disease during a specified time period. [p. 350]

F 27. Herd immunity must be 100% to confer protection to a group. [p. 317]

Multiple choice questions:

1. A person with an inapparent infection: [p. 343]
   *A. Can transmit the infection to others
   B. Is a danger to family members but not to others in the community
   C. Never develops antibodies
   D. Is of no epidemiologic importance

2. You have just finished administering a food/drink questionnaire to ill and non-ill participants in a Minnesota summer picnic party. The ill individuals developed moderate to severe diarrhea 16–46 hours after the picnic. Six persons experienced vomiting. The following data were collected:

	ATE Number of people			DID NOT EAT Number of people		
Food item	Ill	Not ill	Total	Ill	Not ill	Total
Hot dogs	40	30	70	10	20	30
Hamburgers	32	8	40	20	40	60
Potato salad	45	25	70	15	25	40
Ice cream	48	12	60	2	38	40
Lemonade	20	40	60	20	20	40

   Which food item appears to be the most probable vehicle for the salmonella (agent) infection associated with the illness? [p. 346]
   A. Hot dogs
   B. Hamburgers
   C. Potato salad
   *D. Ice cream
   E. Lemonade

Questions 3–5: In two communities of similar size and age structure (A and B), there were outbreaks of viral illnesses (virus A in community A, and virus B in community B) that were each traced back to a single source. Exposure to these viruses in each community confers permanent immunity. In community A, 200 susceptible people were exposed, 150 people were infected, 75 people became ill, and 40 people died. In community B, pathogenicity was 40%, infectivity was 90%, and virulence was 60%. Circle the best response:

3. Which virus had the greatest **infectivity**? [p. 337]
   A. Virus A
   *B. Virus B
   C. Both A and B were equal.

4. Which virus was most **pathogenic**? [p. 337]
   *A. Virus A
   B. Virus B
   C. Both A and B were equal.

5. Which virus was most **virulent**? [p. 338]
   A. Virus A
   *B. Virus B
   C. Both A and B were equal.

6. There are several sources of water that supply Community A. There has been an outbreak of disease X, and it is unknown which source is responsible. The best evidence to determine which suspected water supply is responsible is: [pp. 345–346]
   A. The identity of the water supply providing water to the largest proportion of cases
   B. The relationship between quantity of water consumed and the severity of attack for each individual
   C. The identity of the water supply that has the greatest opportunity for contamination during the epidemic
   *D. The attack rates for disease X in those who did and did not drink from each water supply

7. The Centers for Disease Control and Prevention publish an article concerning the high rate of foot fungal disease in New Orleans. The article explains that there has been a high rate of foot fungal disease in New Orleans for decades. Foot fungal disease in New Orleans is best described as: [p. 365]
   A. Epidemic
   *B. Endemic
   C. Incident
   D. Pathogenic

8. An attack rate is an alternative incidence rate that is used when: [p. 345]
   A. Describing the occurrence of foodborne illness or infectious diseases

B. The population at risk increases greatly over a short time period
C. The disease rapidly follows the exposure during a fixed time period
*D. All of the above

9. An important point about the agent-host-environment model (the epidemiologic triangle) of epidemiologic investigation is that: [pp. 335–341]
   A. The agent is not as important a factor in disease causality as the host or the environment.
   *B. Diseases are multicausal.
   C. It is necessary that the agent be linked to both the host, and the environment and that the agent be present in every case of the disease.
   D. In order to prove causality, which is a difficult task, the researcher must prove that the agent, host, and environmental factors under investigation are both necessary and sufficient to cause the disease being studied.

10. The table below shows the mumps experience of children in 390 families exposed to mumps by a primary case within the family:

Age in years	Population Total	No. susceptible before primary cases occurred	Cases Primary	Secondary
2–4	300	250	100	50
5–9	450	420	204	87
10–19	152	84	25	15

The secondary attack rate among children aged two to four years is: [pp. 347–348]
A. 18%
B. 20%
*C. 33%
D. 50%
E. 60%

[(150 – 100)/(250 – 100) x 100]

Questions 11–14: An outbreak of salmonellosis occurred after an epidemiology department luncheon, which was attended by 485 faculty and staff. Assume everyone ate the same food items. Sixty-five people had fever and diarrhea, five of whom were severely affected. Subsequent laboratory tests on everyone who attended the luncheon revealed an additional 72 cases. [p. 347]

11. The infectivity of salmonellosis was:
    A. 13.4%
    B. 47.4%
    *C. 28.2%
    D. 7.7%
    E. Cannot be calculated from this information

12. The pathogenicity of salmonellosis was:
    A. 13.4%
    *B. 47.4%
    C. 28.2%
    D. 7.7%
    E. Cannot be calculated from this information

13. The virulence of salmonellosis was:
    A. 13.4%
    B. 47.4%
    C. 28.2%
    *D. 7.7%
    E. Cannot be calculated from this information

14. The secondary attack rate of salmonellosis was:
    A. 13.4%
    B. 47.4%
    C. 28.2%
    D. 7.7%
    *E. Cannot be calculated from this information

15. What factors comprise the epidemiologic triangle? [p. 334]
    A. Agent
    B. Host
    C. Environment
    *D. All of the above
    E. A and B only

16. Someone suggests immunization as a means of reducing disease, specifically the feared UJ (uderlinger jacamoodi). What part of the disease cycle is he or she trying to affect? [p. 340]
    *A. Host
    B. Fomites
    C. Vector
    D. Vehicle
    E. Environment

17. Host factors in the causation of disease include: [p. 340]
    A. Temperature and humidity
    B. Chemicals in the air, water, or food.
    *C. Genetic factors
    D. Altitude
    E. All of the above

18. The following disease shows a low subclinical/clinical ratio: [p. 345]
    A. Polio
    B. Epstein-Barr
    C. Hepatitis A in young children
    D. Measles
    *E. A, B, and C

19. The public health officer from Long Beach complains to you about the dread "Pacific Pox." He says, "If people catch the Pox, they suddenly get the urge to dance in the sand and fall dead on the beach within the hour." There are no survivors to interview so you deduce: [p. 349]
    A. The incidence rate of the Pox must be high.
    B. The prevalence of the Pox must be high.
    C. The infectivity of the Pox must be high.
    *D. The case fatality rate of the Pox must be high.
    E. All of the above

20. Attack rate is: [p. 346]
    A. $\dfrac{\text{number of persons who ate a specific food and became ill}}{\text{total number of persons who ate the specific food}}$
    B. $\dfrac{\text{total number of persons who ate a specific food}}{\text{number of persons who did not become ill}}$
    C. Similar to the incidence rate of a disease of short duration
    D. Same as secular trend
    *E. Both A and C

21. In a hypothetical study on rabies in veterinary workers (Spot, 1988), it was found that rabies was almost always fatal. This refers to: [p. 338]
    A. Toxigenicity
    B. Antigenicity
    *C. Virulence
    D. Infectivity

22. Schistosomiasis is an example of: [p. 357]
    A. Chemical agents—carcinogen
    *B. Biological agents—helminth
    C. Allergens—pollen
    D. Physical energy—ionizing radiation

23. Which of the following examples involves indirect transmission of disease? [p. 345]
    A. Malaria
    B. Needle sticks
    C. AIDS
    D. Pneumoconiosis
    *E. A and B

24. The site where a disease enters the body is the: [p. 342]
    A. Reservoir
    *B. Portal of entry
    C. Vehicle
    D. Portal of exit

Essay questions:

1. Disease X is one that often results in severe illness, but never is fatal. On March 21, 1990, 30 students developed disease X among all students enrolled in an introductory epidemiology course at a university. (Assume all epidemiology students were exposed to the index case, the instructor.) Through antibody titers we were able to determine the following: [p. 338]

# of exposed students not infected	40
# of exposed students with subclinical infection	10
# of exposed students with mild symptoms	10
# of exposed students with moderate symptoms	10
# of exposed students with severe symptoms	10

    Using your knowledge of infectious disease epidemiology, **quantify** the pattern of disease X in this group; i.e., what are the infectivity, pathogenicity, and virulence of disease X? [infectivity = 40/80; pathogenicity = 30/40; virulence = 10/30]

2. Imagine you are the State Epidemiologist. Sixty cases of salmonella were reported to you in the last two weeks. Describe how the iceberg model of disease relates to whether this potential disease outbreak needs to be investigated. [p. 344]

Chapter 12: Epidemiologic Aspects of Work and the Environment (pp. 377–406)

Multiple choice questions:

1. One must use care in interpreting occupational differences in morbidity and mortality because: [p. 381]
   * A. Good health status may be a factor for selection into a job.
   B. Occupations involving physical activity tend to cause heart attacks among older workers.
   C. Occupational stress, even in extreme situations, is difficult to quantify.
   D. A, B and C

2. Angiosarcoma of the liver has been associated with: [p. 386]
   A. Pesticides from the organochloride family
   B. Asbestos
   C. Metallic compounds
   * D. Vinyl chloride

3. A sentinel health event refers to: [p. 392]
   A. The correlation between daily mortality and increased air pollution
   B. The nuclear plant accident in Chernobyl, Ukraine
   * C. The cases of unnecessary workplace diseases that serve as warning signals
   D. None of the above

4. Exposure to electric and magnetic fields has been linked to: [p. 389]
   * A. Childhood leukemia risk
   B. Lung cancer
   C. Central nervous system damage
   D. All of the above

5. The healthy worker effect refers to the observation that: [p. 381]
   A. Exercise on the job causes workers to become healthy and gain years of life.
   * B. Healthy persons are more likely to gain employment than unhealthy persons.
   C. Unemployed persons tend to have lower mortality than employed persons.
   D. All of the above

6. A situation in which the combined effect of several exposures is greater than the sum of the individual effects: [p. 384]
   A. Threshold
   B. Latency
   * C. Synergism
   D. None of the above

7. The lowest dose at which a particular response may occur: [p. 383]
   * A. Threshold
   B. Latency
   C. Synergism
   D. None of the above

8. The time period between initial exposure and a measurable response: [p. 384]
   A. Threshold
   * B. Latency
   C. Synergism
   D. None of the above

9. It has been suggested that occupational exposure to benzene in the petroleum industry increases the risk of developing leukemia. The levels of benzene to which workers in this industry have been exposed were high from 1940 to 1970, but since 1970 have been significantly reduced.

   What kind of study design, using petroleum workers, would provide the most useful information on whether benzene affects incidence rates

of leukemia in these industries? (You may assume that records of individual worker assignments to jobs involving benzene exposure have been maintained by the industry.) Circle the best response. [p. 379]
A. Experimental
*B. Retrospective cohort
C. Prospective cohort
D. Case-control
E. Cross-sectional

Essay questions:

1. Recently two follow-up studies of mortality among licensed pesticide applicators were published in the occupational health literature. One study from Florida found an overall standardized mortality ratio (SMR) = 1.80 and excess deaths due to leukemia, cancers of the brain, and lung cancer. A second study, based in Iowa, found an overall SMR = 1.20 and an elevated SMR for lung cancer only. The mortality statistics in each respective state were used for comparison purposes.
   A. Is there reason for concern? Why or why not? [pp. 101–102]
   [Yes, because both SMRs are elevated.]
   B. Why do you think that there was an elevated SMR for only one specific cause of death in Iowa? Knowing that applicators in both states use similar chemicals in their work, do you think that pesticide workers in Florida should be concerned that they may be at higher risk than their colleagues in Iowa? [p. 382]
   [Although several explanations may be advanced, the results may also be spurious.]

2. Investigators conducted a study regarding the effects of water pollution and peptic ulcer disease and obtained the following data: [Review Chapter 3, pp. 72–74]

   A population of 9,000 men and women, aged 45, were examined on January 1, 1985. Of these people, 6,000 were exposed to toxins in the local water supply and 3,000 were not. At the time of this exam, 90 cases of peptic ulcer disease were discovered; 60 of these cases were among those exposed to toxins in their local water.

   All the people at the initial exam who were free from peptic ulcer disease were followed with repeat exams over the following year. This study revealed 268 new cases in the total group; of these, 238 cases were among those exposed to toxins in their local water.

   Calculate the **prevalence** per 1,000 people of peptic ulcer disease on January 1, 1986:

   Among the exposed: (60+238)/6000 x 1000 = 49.7/1000

   Among the non-exposed: (30+30)/3000 x 1000 = 20/1000

   Calculate the 1985 **incidence** rate/1,000 people of peptic ulcer disease:

   Among the exposed: 238/5940 x 1000 = 40.1/1000/yr.

   Among the non-exposed: 30/2970 x 1000 = 10.1/1000/yr.

   In the total sample: 268/8910 x 1000 = 30.1/1000/yr.

Chapter 13: Molecular and Genetic Epidemiology (pp. 407–440)

Classroom exercise: Assign the students to search the literature for a recent article on the genetic epidemiology of any disease of interest (preferably a case-control study). Have them retrieve the article, read it, and see if it contains information to answer the following:
  A. What is the nature of the genetic marker (a candidate gene, anonymous DNA marker, etc.)?
  B. Is the genetic marker known to be functionally significant?
  C. What is the frequency of the genetic marker among the controls?
  D. Does the marker vary by race or ethnicity, and, if so, are the study groups comparable?

1. One of the potential limitations of case-control studies of the biological basis of disease is that the disease process may alter the exposure of interest. Is that a concern for germline DNA?

    Answer: No. Our germline DNA does not change. We may acquire mutations in specific tissues, but collection of a blood sample for extraction of DNA will result in the procurement of constitutional DNA.

2. For some rare autosomal dominant diseases, it is possible that the dominant homozygote has never been seen. One reason is that the fetus with this genotype may die early in development and be spontaneously aborted. In fact, roughly 25% of all women will have a pregnancy end in spontaneous abortion at some point in their life. Consider a situation in which:

    Q/Q dies as an early fetus
    Q/q lives to reproduce but is unaffected
    q/q lives and is unaffected

    What genotypes are possible among live-born children of the mating Q/q X Q/q?

    Answer: ¼ of the potential offspring will be Q/Q and die in utero. Therefore, only Q/q and q/q will be observed. ⅔ will be Q/q and ⅓ will be q/q.

3. Cancer of the kidney constitutes about 2% of all human cancer, and renal cell carcinoma comprises about 85% of all kidney cancers. Although the etiology is largely unknown, a quick review of the literature reveals nearly 30 case reports of familial aggregates. Can one conclude that renal cell carcinoma is hereditary?

    Answer: No. There may be a hereditary component, but common environmental exposure must be considered, as well as the role of chance.

4. Family history of disease is often used as a surrogate marker of genetic susceptibility. For a common disease with a late and variable age at onset, what two factors play a significant role in your interpretation of a case-control study of family history?

    Answer: The number of relatives at risk in the two study groups, and the corresponding ages of the relatives.

5. A segregation analysis of a large set of randomly selected families suggests weak evidence for a genetic influence on obesity. The investigators split their families into two groups, based on the median age of the probands. Results indicate a substantial genetic influence on obesity in the late-onset group of families, but no significant genetic influence on the early-onset group of families. You intend to map the gene (or genes) that influence risk of obesity. Would you measure risk factors on family members, and, if so, what?

6. Genetic linkage studies can either be based on a model of inheritance or parameter free. For the former, one needs to know the mode of inheritance and the penetrance (age-risk function). What are the three ways that penetrance values can be obtained for presumed genetic susceptibles?

Answer: Perform a segregation analysis; use values from a published segregation analysis; make them up.

What are the options for non-susceptibles?

Answer: Use population rates of disease or segregation analysis.

7. Twelve families are selected for a genetic linkage study because of a high prevalence of disease. A genome screen is performed, using anonymous DNA markers on all autosomes. Significant evidence for linkage is observed to a marker on chromosome 2 (D2S123) in four families. The LOD score for the remaining families at this locus is significantly negative. How do you interpret this finding?

Answer: There is likely to be genetic heterogeneity—different genes exist—and further research is needed to identify remaining candidate regions.

8. You are interested in identifying the role of genetic factors in alcoholism. A case-control study is done of alcoholics and age- and sex-matched controls. DNA is obtained and the alcohol dehydrogenase three gene is analyzed for a common genetic polymorphism. The frequency of the polymorphism is found to be significantly more common among cases than controls. The polymorphism results in a silent amino acid substitution, and functional studies indicate that the variant and the normal allele have similar activity. How do you interpret your finding?

Answer: A number of possibilities should be explored. If the allele frequency differs by race and ethnicity, the study groups should be examined for comparability (confounding). It may also be that the genetic variant under study is simply linked (linkage disequilibrium) to a functional mutation either in another exon, or in some part of the gene that regulates transcription (enhancer or promoter region). Finally, one must acknowledge that the findings could simply reflect chance.

Chapter 14: Psychologic, Behavioral, and Social Epidemiology (pp. 441–475)

Multiple choice questions:

1. Psychosocial epidemiology deals with the health effects of: [p. 444]
   A. Stress
   B. Culture
   C. Personal behavior
   D. Social factors
   *E. All of the above

2. Researchers (e.g., Fox) have concluded that there is an absence of an association between cancer outcomes and: [p. 467]
   A. Stress
   B. Depressed mood
   C. Psychosis
   D. Bereavement
   *E. All of the above

3. Sociocultural influences on health include: [p. 461]
   A. Specific behaviors associated with daily living
   B. Mediation of stress exposure
   C. Health services utilization
   *D. All of the above

4. Personal behavior and lifestyle factors in health do not include: [pp. 454–461]
   *A. Social support
   B. Alcohol consumption
   C. Dietary practices
   D. Lack of exercise

5. Which of the following statements describes the person-environment fit model? [p. 448]
   A. Discrepancy between husband and wife in social and educational status
   *B. Goodness of fit between the characteristics of the person and environment
   C. Stressors that result from the happenings in one's existence
   D. None of the above

6. Which of the following statements describes life events? [p. 449]
   A. Discrepancy between husband and wife in social and educational status
   B. Goodness of fit between the characteristics of the person and environment
   *C. Stressors that result from the happenings in one's existence
   D. None of the above

7. Selye's concept of the general adaptation syndrome **did not include:** [p. 446]
   A. Alarm reaction
   *B. Stage of recovery
   C. Stage of resistance
   D. Stage of exhaustion

8. Examples of social incongruity include: [p. 447]
   A. Discrepancy between parents in social status
   B. Discrepancy between generations, e.g., fathers and sons
   C. Changes from rural to urban residence
   *D. All of the above

9. The most important methodological problems in the measurement of life events are: [p. 450]
   A. Subject's recall ability
   B. Reliability of measurement
   C. Memory biases
   *D. A, B, and C
   E. Number of items in the questionnaire

10. The type A behavior pattern is hypothesized to be a risk factor for: [p. 451]
    A. Chronic obstructive pulmonary disease
    *B. Coronary heart disease
    C. Rheumatoid arthritis
    D. All of the above

11. Which of the following conditions would not be likely to be considered a Western or way-of-life disease? [p. 458]
    *A. Bacterial infection
    B. Diverticular disease
    C. Obesity
    D. Diabetes
    E. Gallbladder disease

Essay questions:

1. Describe how the diet-heart hypothesis represents a multifactorial model for the etiology of coronary heart disease. In what way is the diet-heart hypothesis inconsistent with the epidemiologic triangle? [p. 460]

2. Discuss the association between sedentary lifestyle and heart disease. Be sure to cite examples of specific research studies. [p. 461]

3. What are some of the possible associations between personality and smoking? What kinds of study designs might be utilized to investigate these hypothesized associations? [p. 467]